BETH

A STORY OF POSTPARTUM PSYCHOSIS

By

Shirley Cervene Halvorson

ISBN: 1-4140-3110-6 (e-book)
ISBN: 1-4140-3111-4 (Paperback)
ISBN: 1-4140-3112-2 (Dust Jacket)

Library of Congress Control Number: 2004090210

This book is printed on acid-free paper.

Printed in the United States of America
Bloomington, IN

1stBooks – rev. 01/23/04

Acknowledgements

Special thanks go to Jane Honikman, founder of Postpartum Support International, for her guidance and loving care, and to Dr. Cort Pedersen, M.D., UNC-CH, School of Medicine, for his encouragement.

Thanks also to those who serve new mothers everywhere.

Dedication

Especially to Beth Ellen Halvorson Flack, loving daughter, wife, and sister, and the reason for this publication.

and

to my dear patient husband, Dave, our sons, Gary, Jim, and Michael and our grandson, Kyle.

Preface

This book is written to share my experience with postpartum psychosis, illustrate some of the risk factors and behaviors found in postpartum mental illness, and reassure all those who suffer from a postpartum disorder that they will be able to find help. There is no need for new mothers or babies to die when such help is now available.

This story is not an ending but a beginning of new attitudes, new research and literature, and new methods of treatment due to mothers like Beth who have paved the way to making an illness both treatable and temporary.

The Mission

It was in 1986 when I was first exposed to the world of postpartum depression, which took the form of postpartum psychosis in our daughter, Beth, following the birth of her first child. At that time, no one seemed to have a name for this phenomenon or was even willing to admit there was a connection between birth and depression, anxiety, or psychosis. This experience would cause me great feelings of inadequacy and helplessness when Beth committed suicide five months later.

Even though she committed suicide, her death was actually caused by postpartum psychosis, along with a lack of medical knowledge available at that time. We now know that postpartum mental illnesses are temporary and treatable. And we have literature and new medications to help. Good therapy is available. But this took many years, and I searched valiantly for answers wherever I could.

As an inquiring person, and because my daughter endured great emotional pain, I started looking for material to explain why she died and what caused it. I finally came across a book called <u>The New Mother Syndrome</u>, by Carol Dix. It seemed to explain some of what we saw in Beth. Although the doctor refused to read it, the information at the back of that book gave me contact information for people who were better acquainted with the subject.

After the suicide, I felt an urgency to know all I could about why Beth died and what caused it. I swore if I found out some way to help even one woman, it would be worth the time and effort. I wrote several letters to the organizations listed in Dix's book and also to Dr. James A. Hamilton of California. He promptly answered my request to find helpful groups in the United States.

Dr. James A. Hamilton, MD gave me the names of Jane Honikman and Nancy Berchtold. Jane had a support group in California, and Nancy had one in Pennsylvania. Both were highly recommended, and they were the only two known support groups in the country!

I began a correspondence with Nancy, who had a small amount of information on what they called postpartum depression. Nancy had suffered from psychosis after her daughter was born, and she seemed quite knowledgeable. She called me, wrote to me, and sent me a few materials. I was hungry to know more.

Nancy invited me and my husband, Dave, to attend a conference in Princeton, NJ the next summer, in 1987. We attended and met such wonderful people who also had personal experiences with postpartum depression or psychosis. They were warm and kind, and the conference turned out to be the beginning of the two groups I would become involved with: Depression After Delivery, Inc. (DAD) and Postpartum Support International (PSI).

I had the opportunity to meet Jane Honikman, founder of Postpartum Support International (PSI), and Dr. James Hamilton, who was a sort of grandfather and medical expert to both organizations. It was a wonderful experience, and it whet my appetite to learn more. I felt these two organizations could help me immeasurably. They have done just that.

My first job was as a contact person for DAD (Nancy Berchtold's now national organization). I was also on the Board of Directors from North Carolina. I took calls from new mothers everywhere that had postpartum problems and didn't know where to turn. It was amazing and scary! What if I said the wrong thing? Would I cause more severe problems? What to say or do? I learned through these conversations.

Depression After Delivery is a grassroots telephone support group with a free phone line. They dispense materials to new mothers and professionals, and they maintain telephone contact all over the

United States. Most of the contact people were young mothers who had experienced postpartum depression. DAD provided workshops and conferences where they stressed education, information, support and referrals as major goals. I believe education is primary and tried to attend all of them. As a teacher, I realized I could really be of help. I learned much from the new mothers at the workshops and within DAD, as well as from those I spoke to on the telephone. An organizational newsletter was sent to all members, and it always included a personal experience and recovery from postpartum depression or anxiety.

It wasn't long before conferences were offered jointly by DAD and PSI. They were wonderful and provided a much-needed education to anyone interested, including professionals and new mothers. My husband Dave and I traveled all over the country and Canada to become acquainted with survivors of postpartum disorders, medical doctors, and other professionals who were currently working on "getting the word out."

We joined PSI as well, and gained more knowledge and friendship. Postpartum Support International extends to all countries and provides information, educational opportunities, training, and certification. Postpartum Support International sends a member newsletter, maintains a lending library with information about starting support groups, supports ongoing research, and provides state coordinators. Both DAD, Inc. and PSI maintain excellent web sites.

Presently, I am the North Carolina Coordinator for PSI, and also president of my own group, North Carolina Depression After Delivery.

Little by little, research has been done and books have been and are being written in the field of postpartum disorders. PSI sponsors annual and ongoing conferences. Over the years, I have "beat the bushes" for helpers, and those who need help are finding us. I have read extensively and pursued all possible educational avenues. My rewards have been great! Many new mothers and families have contacted me by phone or e-mail for help over the years.

Today, sixteen years later, there is no need for any woman to suffer any form of postpartum depression. The educational materials, research, new medicines, and informed persons are available to all who seek them.

I have learned and gone forward, in spite of my loss. My church friends refer to my postpartum depression work as a "special ministry." It is heartwarming to see that others have dedicated themselves to future work in the area of postpartum disorders and to see that they are very committed to this. It is especially so with those who have lost someone or suffered personally. My HOPE is still the same: if I can help one mother, it will be worth every minute of my time. My daughter would be proud!

Chapter 1
A Little Bit About Beth

Beth Ellen Halvorson was born in Elmer, NJ in 1961. She was a beautiful little girl with dark hair and blue eyes, and she was an immediate joy to us all. After three wonderful boys, we now had our girl. It was soon after the birth that she became very ill for the first year. Once diagnosed with celiac syndrome, and after a "near death scare," we were able to get her on a proper diet, and things were much better from then on. At one point, I had a sign stitched to her jacket so our neighbors would not give her cookies or crackers. She thought it was a great idea, and it worked!

Beth was a very pretty baby and became a lovely young lady with dark brown hair, green eyes, and was all of 5 feet, 3 inches and 105 pounds. She was pleased to be one inch taller than I was. She was always confident, outgoing, fun-loving and exuberant about life. Her smile was contagious.

She was loved so much by the boys that they dubbed her "Beth Ellen Sweetie Pie." They took her everywhere, volunteered to feed her, and helped her with whatever she needed. But she was very independent and tried to be grown up, like she felt they were. And she grew into a perfect tomboy, climbing trees and insisting, "Mom, I have to have some 'boy shoes' to climb the pussy willows in the back!" She got her shoes, and loved them.

She was the adopted "congregational baby" in our church. I was the organist, so I watched as she was spoiled and entertained by other families. She learned German words from many of our members, was given treats, and had lots of hugs and shoulder rides. She thoroughly enjoyed it. As she grew in the church, she became spiritually involved. On Good Friday, she was always in tears. The only Good Friday Service she ever missed was the one right before her death. Her devotion to the Lord served her well all of her life.

For many years, I shopped in the same grocery store and took Beth along. She busied herself by talking to people and then reporting what they had to say back to me; she was about three years old at that time. She connected with people easily and asked many questions, especially about handicapped people. She was so empathetic, and people seem to appreciate her interest.

I had always been told there was no ladies' room in that store. Beth was going through a phase of extreme interest in different bathrooms. We always said she was toilet trained on a trip to Florida because she wanted to see new bathrooms. Once I told her we had to hurry because there was no bathroom in the store. She said, "Sure there is, Mommy!" I protested. "Come with me," she pointed to the back. Sure enough, she took me up a flight of stairs and there was a huge bathroom and sitting room. "See, I told you, Mommy," she said. I was amazed at how resourceful a little three-year-old child can be.

She went through the usual dancing, piano, and clarinet lessons parents are so good at cramming down their children's throats. But she actually got up early and practiced before school and was quite proficient at all three. When she tripped on the rug or her own feet, we used to tease her about being a klutz and ask her, "Are you really a ballet student?" She would laugh at that. The piano lessons continued until about eighth grade, and she was very good. I always told her I didn't like "Fur Elise", a certain piece of music that I never wanted for my own piano lessons. I hoped she wouldn't play it either. Then one day she walked in with it in her hands. "Guess what I got assigned for my lesson this week?" It was "Fur Elise". We had a few laughs and I knew she purposely asked for it. We also did a few duets together.

The clarinet was her pride and joy, and she achieved prominence in high school band, sitting first chair. She even spent some time as a "flag girl" for the band. It was my mistake to grant her permission to try out her first year. I had no idea she would be so good and be accepted. This meant buying a uniform, boots, hat and other paraphernalia. I was so proud, I was glad to spend the money.

She readily volunteered me for things like teaching music at a Scout meeting to playing for members of her concert band for solos. Music often brought her friends into the house, and she asked me to play for them to sing along.

Going to the Senior Center to entertain was a true love for her, and she showed it by learning a song or a dance to perform. Well in advance of these Senior Center trips, she would say, "Guess what, Mom? I learned a new song to sing (or a dance, or poem), and I want to go with you to the Senior Center this month. May I please go?" She visited easily with the older people, and they enjoyed her.

She became an avid reader, perhaps due to her brother, Mike, who took her to the library regularly from the time she could walk that far. He had a great love for reading. She developed the same love. Her brother, Gary, introduced art. He painted and exhibited his paintings and drawings from his art class on our family room bulletin board wall. She became a lover of sports, especially swimming, through Jim, our middle son. All of them swam on a team, but Jim was so gung-ho that she asked to be on the team when she was five years old. And she was pretty good.

Since we regularly attended the theater, this became of particular importance to Beth. She loved attending plays, concerts, and the ballet as a family.

She became acquainted with new ideas when she attended a Friend's School with me where I taught music. Her brother, Gary, attended the school, and he introduced her to people of all races, religions and countries. She preferred spending her time with the kindergarten class and the black teacher (Teacher Doris) who played the piano.

One of her best friends there was a little Indian girl named Arun. Arun's mother was a teacher and her older sister was in my class. They were from India and taught us about that culture, cooking, hospitality, and friendship. Beth was impressed by the size of Arun's huge birthday party. It is an Indian custom to invite the whole town, we discovered.

She became quite an advocate for her black friends, Indian friends, and other friends when she felt they were being threatened. She really kept us on our toes, we always wondered what was going to happen next. I believe she was the first child in our southern Texas neighborhood to invite a black friend to her house for a birthday party.

The teen years were the most difficult. Horses were her first love for a while. She got a job through a friend who was working on a ranch. She loved one horse so much she agreed to work for his feed since his owner could not afford it at the time. The ranch had very large racehorses, and I was shocked to find her one afternoon working alone in the barn with this huge black stallion. She had his back hoof pulled up and was digging the dirt out of it. This was also the place where she lost her first contact lens, in the straw, where I had asked her never to wear them. A teen, for sure!

She was "madly in love" with a young man from Texas at one point. She even thought of eloping with him. Then her good sense kicked in. We had recently moved to North Carolina, and Beth was lonely for her friends, although she was happy in school (especially in band).

She spent many hours at the Rescue Squad in High School. She was a good student and loved to help others. She acquired her emergency medical technician certification. She spent many hours in classes, as well as spending time down at the squad. She answered the phones and generally enjoyed the fellowship.

Beth spent a year in nursing school, but felt it was not what she anticipated even though she was an honors student. She came home and tried several jobs, which finally led her to work with computers.

She and Mike were married the following year. They had been dating for nearly four years. Mike was a little older and more established. They were happy, enjoyed each other, and were constantly joking. Her sense of humor never left until the psychosis. **The one thing I miss most is her beautiful smile.**

Chapter 2

A Dream Fulfilled

It was a sunny warm day in the spring of 1986 when I looked up from my desk and saw my 25-year old daughter, Beth, standing shyly at the door. It was so nice to see her looking so happy. I smiled, and she seemed slightly self-conscious about something. School was out for the day, but a few students remained. I motioned her in and wondered why she was there, as it was unusual for her to come to the school. Her huge smile seemed very secretive – like she was up to something. She was!

She was very excited and approached me with a large hug saying, "You're going to be a grandma, Mom!" We hugged, and I dismissed the students. She had been waiting for this day for quite a while. It was a day for celebration! After the initial excitement Beth and I called our homes and arranged for a celebration dinner at the pizza place. Everyone was so happy: Beth, Mike (her husband), Dave (her dad) and me! Finally, I would have a little grandchild right in town, and could see him as often as I liked. Since our other grandchildren lived in Texas, this would be such fun!

What a thrill it was for Beth and Mike to have their dream come true. They had carefully planned the pregnancy after buying a house, decorating it, finding job security, and readied themselves to extend their family. They had been happily married five years. We saw them frequently. Although Beth did not become pregnant immediately, the wait increased the excitement for all of us. I knew she would be a wonderful mother, since she had so much experience with children.

The pregnancy was quite normal–no real problems. But I noticed she was so happy all the time, it seemed unusual. Looking back, I think she was manic. But how do you tell your daughter's doctor that she is "too happy," and why would I even feel this was unusual? Perhaps because most pregnancies bring some discomfort – I know I wasn't happy all the time during my pregnancies. Although I was never able to eliminate the idea that something was not right, I made a conscious decision not to say anything and just be glad things were going so well for her. She carried a large bottle of Rolaids with her and laughed about her indigestion.

I had taken a year's leave of absence from teaching for the following school year, and we spent a lot of time together. We went to the library every week, and Beth was an avid reader and much faster at it than I. We shopped for maternity clothes, discussed baby names, enjoyed lunch together, picked out baby necessities, and planned the baby's room. We talked about a theme for the room, and I grudgingly agreed to make curtains for her. I hate to sew! But I was willing to try. She was always teasing me about it.

"Oh, Mom, you know you can do it. Remember that square dance dress you made in Texas?"

I often made her school clothes when she was younger, usually on demand, and it was always such a struggle. But I always gave in because she was so sincere, saying things like:

"Oh yes, I promise to iron it myself, promise, promise, promise!" or "But I just love this pattern, and I know you can do it. Pleeeze?"

A few weeks later, she called and said she had chosen just the right material and said, "Let's get the curtains made, Mom." Beth had chosen primary colors that would brighten up the room. She had also bought a crib blanket with a large blue elephant in the center with lots of red, yellow, blue and green. She came to "watch" me, and we laughed about our little sewing joke. She wanted things to be just

10

right. She kept me company, and the deed was done. I secretly made a matching quilt and pillow for the crib. She was thrilled! She thanked me over and over and hugged me. She was a super "hugger" and showed love openly and often.

Beth was also the family "glue"! She kept up with the boys regularly on the phone and reminded them of things like, "Don't forget, it is Mom's birthday next week." She made sure she knew what they were doing, and if there was a problem, she usually told me and asked me to call them. They seemed to love her involvement with them, and she seemed to be able to say anything to them without making them upset.

We had made plans to meet for lunch about three weeks before "Kyle" was to be born. I waited and waited. It was not like her to be late, so I was concerned that something awful had happened. Then the phone rang. "Mom, guess where I am? I am in the hospital, and the baby will be born today." I was dumbfounded. She explained, "I went to the doctor this morning, and he accidentally 'broke my water.'"

I was disturbed by this, but let it slip by. I did not like her choice of doctors and knew this one had been chastised in the past by the hospital. "Could you come to the hospital sometime soon?" she asked. Since Mike was already there with her, I waited for awhile. I was very excited, but knew it would be a while before the baby came.

Chapter 3
The Birth

Around 6 o'clock, December 2, 1986, I set off for the hospital. Beth had been in bed since early that morning and was being monitored. She had a band around her belly, and nurses were taking vital signs regularly. Mike's parents were waiting behind a curtained area. She asked me to come in with her. She was so happy! When the labor became intense, she asked me, "Mom, I don't want to hurt your feelings, but would you mind waiting so I can do this with Mike?" I went to sit with Mike's parents. It was around 8 o'clock p.m.

About midnight, I heard her doctor say, "You are not doing enough, and if you don't try harder, I will have to use instruments. Your baby is caught on your pelvic bone." He sounded totally unsympathetic, and he left the room. I could see and hear everything from the corner of the curtain. She was purple by then from pushing so hard. Her doctor encouraged her to begin pushing at least two hours earlier. She was gasping for breath, but I heard her tell Mike she was going to do this by herself and that she didn't want the doctor to use instruments to deliver her baby. No medications were given. I knew it would be difficult, and I was worried. This doctor seemed disinterested by her stress and checked her occasionally but always left the room immediately. The obstetrician offered no words of encouragement.

The doctor remained in the hall where I sought him out about two hours later. I asked him how long he was going to leave her like this. "Oh, about 3 hours," he said. It was now about 3:00 am. Hard labor had begun about 9:00 pm – six hours earlier. She had been in bed since the morning. His lack of caring must have been traumatic to Beth. I felt like slapping him.

I knew Beth would want to do everything she could to keep the baby safe. She often said she wanted everything to be perfect. She would do whatever she was told. This baby meant everything to her. She sang to him, talked to him, and read to him, even before he was born. She laughed about the reading when I asked. She loved children and had taken care of infants and children for many years. She was also a perfectionist.

(*Perfectionism in new mothers can be a risk factor for postpartum depression.*)

But I could not stay any longer. I was extremely discouraged and angry about the doctor's attitude. Since his actions were questionable and lacking in kindness, I became frightened and uneasy. I found it very difficult to see my child suffer and needed to get home and away from this traumatic scene. My own medications were overdue, but I hated to leave. Staying became unbearable. My husband was out of town.

I asked the doctor to let Beth know my reason for leaving and to have her call me when the baby was born. I felt badly that I couldn't stay, but it seemed like she was being tortured.

At about 4:00 am the call came. She was exuberant! I was very relieved that she sounded so well and that it was over. She talked a mile a minute and said, "We have a little boy and named him Kyle Mills. He weighs 7 pounds, 13 ounces." (She was being stitched up at the time.) "He is so beautiful that I don't even care if I have problems with the stitches." She asked if I was alright. She was on "Cloud Nine"! It had been an instrument delivery which, we were to discover later, had caused a great deal of bleeding. I was pleased she was well and happy, and that the baby was fine. I told her how much I loved her. She said, "Mom, can you come to the hospital tomorrow to see Kyle?" Of course I said yes.

Kyle Mill Flack was born on December 3rd, 1968.

(*Excessive bleeding is a contributing factor to Postpartum Psychosis.*)

Chapter 4
The Immediate Aftermath

The following day, I went to the hospital to see Beth and my new little Kyle. She was withdrawn, tired, and uninterested in Kyle. I thought it was just the long labor and delivery, but clearly something was wrong. Her father-in-law was holding the baby when I got there. It is unusual when you willingly give your new baby over to others immediately. He had been there and holding Kyle for over an hour.

She then asked, "Would you like to hold him, Mom?" Of course I did. This behavior continued through the first week. She later came to church with Kyle and wanted me to hold him. I vowed to keep an eye on her when she came home. For some reason, she was trying to avoid holding her baby.

(We now know that this avoidance behavior is part of postpartum psychosis and is usually due to fear of harming the baby.)

I made a point to stop in every day that first week. I could see she was tense. She told me she did not sleep well and said she was up checking on the baby all night. She became agitated. She stood in the kitchen with clenched fists on about the third day and said, "Mom, when will this stop? I feel terrible!" I thought it was "baby blues" at first, but could see it was more serious. It frightened both of us, and we didn't understand what was happening. She said, "Why didn't they tell me this could happen when I went to all those classes at the hospital?" I wanted the answer to that question myself. They had both attended birthing classes, but postpartum illnesses were not discussed.

(New mothers need to be educated during pregnancy.)

She became totally frustrated with nursing. I sent a friend to help her, and Beth told my friend, "I wish I could go back 10 months." My friend told me this when she saw me later that day and also said she didn't know the meaning of this statement. I didn't understand it either. It was frightening, and I did not want to think about it. What was the real message? It was about the third day after the delivery.

Dave and I returned to her house that same evening. She felt badly, because she wanted to do everything just right. Her behavior was bizarre; she darted back and forth to the bathroom to use the breast pump while constantly saying "I just can't do this!" She pulled on her shirt while trying to use the breast pump and cried all the while. This was something she would never do in front of her dad. She said she was upset about not being able to breastfeed and was quitting.

Beth told me repeatedly, "I can't feed him!" At first I thought it was because she couldn't see the amount of milk Kyle was consuming. Seeing a bottle of milk disappear is easier, so I suggested she try bottle feeding. She was so obviously depressed, and I began to worry. There seemed nothing I could do but suggest she start using bottles. Perhaps if she saw how much Kyle was drinking, it would help soothe her. She was overly disturbed. I couldn't understand or stop it. She was inconsolable. She began using the bottles the next day.

Dave and I discussed this in the car on the way home, and both of us were confused and very worried. We had never seen her so distressed before.

On the fifth day, she discovered she was packed full of gauze from the excessive bleeding during the birth. She phoned me to tell me all about it. The doctor had not even told her about the gauze, and she discovered it and removed it. She said, "I am so mad at my doctor for not even telling me about this gauze, I am done with him. I am never going back to him." She was very angry. I began to wonder about a possible infection. I planned to see her every day until I found out what was wrong.

I was late arriving the seventh day, exactly one week from the birth. As I was coming up the steps to the little rancher, I saw her through the glass door sitting on the couch, staring into space. Tears were streaming down her face. She seemed listless but glad to see me, if only to tell me what was going on. All I could think of was a picture I had seen of someone in a catatonic state, staring into nothingness. I asked, "What is wrong, Honey?" She said, "Everything!" The crying became loud and panicky. It slowed down a little when she was assured I wouldn't leave. I quickly ducked into the bedroom and saw that Kyle was asleep and well. She seemed glad and relieved to see me.

It was obvious that she was seriously depressed, and it seemed to be worse than any depression I had ever seen. It was scary! Such a lot of suffering, and I could do nothing! I had seen depression many times and recognized the symptoms, but had never seen anyone in her condition. She was slow of speech. She had become very pale and was unaware of her surroundings. Confusion was evident. She begged me to take Kyle and keep him. She said, "I can't take care of him. I don't know how to feed him." Convinced she could not take care of him, she pleaded, "Mom, you know how to take care of Kyle, and I can't do it." She was crying harder. "I want you to keep him!" She was begging me. I was stunned and unsure what she meant. She clarified it by saying she had to get him out of the house, and I should be his mother. She said, "Mom, you have to take him home with you!" She was fearful for him, or maybe, herself!

I was now in a quandary! I thought if I really took Kyle, it may push her into a suicide, because she was no longer needed. On the other hand, if I didn't take him, she may harm him and herself. Whatever I said would have to be weighed carefully, and I felt the need to be in control of my emotions and the situation. Could I do this? I had to do something! It seemed dangerous to leave her alone with Kyle. There was no question about my leaving–I knew I could not. It was obvious she needed professional help. I was extremely frightened, but I remained calm, at least on the outside. I was sitting with my arm around her, trying to soothe her. Over and over she talked about not being able to feed him properly. I promised to help her.

(Confusion, inability to cope, depression, hopelessness, helplessness – all are part of postpartum mood disorders.)

I tried to find out if she had eaten lunch, but she didn't remember. I brought her some iced tea. She could barely hold it and seemed not to realize she had a glass in her hand. When she did not drink, I took it from her. She didn't seem to realize that it was no longer in her hand. The crying had stopped momentarily. She was sitting on the couch just as she had been when I arrived. She began to sob again and said, "I did something to Kyle today that I shouldn't have done. But I can't tell you. Mike got mad at me when I told him." "Is he alright?" I asked. I suddenly became aware that I may have missed something when I checked on him. "Yes, Mom. I didn't hurt him, and he is sleeping in the crib." She kept sobbing and making irrational statements, and it made me angry at myself for not recognizing her detachment from the real world earlier. He was fine when I looked in on him again.

It is extremely difficult to recognize irrational statements if you don't expect them. It had taken me much too long to understand what was happening. I was trying to get enough sense of the entire situation to be able to contact a medical professional. It seemed necessary to question her. I tried to mentally file those characteristics that were unusual and frightening, so I could help the doctor. Much of what she said did not make any sense. It was unbelievable that this could be happening!

(*Irrationality is a sign of psychosis.*)

What triggered the mood she was in? I asked what had happened.

"My obstetrician's office called."

I asked, "Why did he call? And what was said?"

Beth replied, "The nurse said I should be grateful to have a live baby, because everyone was not so lucky, and to get down on my knees and 'pray that Devil out of my house.'"

Beth had not contacted his office herself, so did not understand the reason she was called. She was very emotional, so I had trouble understanding all of this. Because she was not rational earlier, I began to doubt the truth of what she said. But I later found out she understood exactly. The nurse who called her verified the conversation.

Beth's speech was slowing. The crying stopped. She was very tired. I realized her dependence on me when she stated, "Mom, you are the only one I trust." She didn't want me to call Mike, because he had been there earlier. She was not going to bother him at work. She leaned against me–her way of saying, "Take care of me." I was frightened, worried, and very angry, and reviled this obstetrician and his staff! I realized someone had to take care of her. She never left the couch. She had become totally dysfunctional, just sitting and unaware of herself–unable to do anything on her own. SHE NEEDED HELP IMMEDIATELY!

I began to try and sort it all out and decide what to do. My mind was asking, "What professional would say something like, 'the devil is in your house,' etc?" I was stunned. I was to learn later that her friend, Linda, had been there in the morning. When Linda discovered that Beth could not even pour the formula into a bottle, she completed the task for Beth. Then Linda called Beth's doctor to let them know there was a severe problem. This was their answer to Linda's phone call – a frightening phone call to an unknowing Beth!

Beth told me, "I tried to kill myself but it didn't work." As frightening as that was, I remained as calm as possible. Fortunately, I have lived through a lot of emergencies with four children. But never like this! My stomach was protesting loudly, and my brain was telling me to keep calm in spite of terrible fear. I sat down across from Beth.

"What did you do?" I asked.

"I tried to smother myself with a pillow."

"What made you stop?"

"I couldn't breathe."

All of this was told in an almost inaudible voice. This was definitely not a rational statement. It was terrifying! What was happening? Where was my real daughter? What should I do now?

(Suicide and infanticide are frequently part of postpartum psychosis. Delusions and hallucinations are part of it, too.)

I knew Beth should see a psychiatrist immediately, but I decided to call the obstetrician first from her house, if only to check the possibility of what he could do to help. During all of this, she had not moved from the couch. I didn't know how much she understood, but I did know she trusted me. I had to admit that I wanted to know if the obstetrician really would try to help.

He answered the phone, and I identified myself as Beth Flack's mother.

He immediately said, "I understand you have a little problem, but I can't do anything about that. You will have to get a psychiatrist."

I decided to push.

"Who should I call?"

"Oh, they are all good."

"What about Dr. Jones?"

"Oh, yes, he is fine."

"Will you call him, or should I call?"

"Oh no, you call him. Just tell him I sent you."

I felt the obstetrician was an absolute dead end. It was obvious he did not want to be involved. If he really wanted to help, he would have suggested a psychiatrist. It was up to me to get help. If only I had some kind of explanation for all of this.

Chapter 5
Available Help?

Since the obstetrician wished to take no responsibility, I then called a psychiatrist I knew, Dr Jones. Dr. Jones made an appointment for us a few hours later, and I called Mike at work so he could come with us. Mike was relieved to know that something was being done and said, "I'm so glad you are doing something for her." He thanked me and said he would be home immediately. Mike and I took Kyle and Beth to the appointment. After Dr. Jones examined Beth, he came out and said, "Beth has the worst depression and psychosis I have ever seen."

He recommended immediate hospitalization in the psychiatric ward at the hospital. Mike and I would have to take her right away. This made me feel a little better, as someone could keep a suicide watch over her. We took her directly to the hospital. It was so hard for all of us.

We were all standing just inside the locked psychiatric ward doors near the hallway to the rooms. Beth held Kyle lovingly in her arms in the wheelchair when a nurse passed by and almost yelled.

"You cannot have that baby in here! Don't you know any better?"

Then one of the patients approached us, and Beth became very protective of Kyle. She said to me, "Mom, don't let any of these people touch him, they are all crazy!" I assured her it would be alright, and tried to comfort her by taking the responsibility for watching Kyle.

Then I took Kyle, and a nurse took Beth to her room. Mike and I could barely get to the elevator before we collapsed on each other, crying. It is one of the hardest things in the world to lock up your own daughter! It haunted me. Did I do the right thing? Was he a good doctor? How long would she be there? Why didn't I get her there sooner? Perhaps they could have helped her more if she had been brought in earlier. The list of guilt goes on and on.

(In 1986 Postpartum Psychosis was virtually unknown in the United States. Few doctors knew and understood it. Materials were

almost impossible to find. It was during this time period that Depression After Delivery and Postpartum Support International were born. Unfortunately, they were not there in time for Beth.)

Chapter 6

The Local Hospital

I know some hospitals and some psychiatrists are good. But I still didn't want to leave my only daughter, who needed me, in such a place.

Our hospital served the community. It was a fairly large eight-story building that was gray-colored but pleasant. On the seventh floor, they had the psychiatric wards. These were locked, and there was a nurses' station, behind glass, where you could ask for entrance. You were not always granted entrance.

Part of this area was designated for teens and others with severe drug and behavioral problems. I had been there before to see one of my former students who had become suicidal.

The other part of the floor housed people with different kinds of mental illness, such as manic-depressives, schizophrenics, clinically depressed, etc. This was the part Beth was housed in.

There was a television room near the nurses' desk. Most of the sleeping area had two beds per room. A few rooms were set aside for art therapy and meetings. There was another area, which I could not see, where some patients were locked in solitude. Beth told me of this locked area. There was a tiny room near the entrance where you could sit a few minutes if you were visiting a patient – kind of a vestibule. It was all quite austere and cold. I could never feel comfortable there and felt I was being observed constantly. Actually, I *was* being observed, I discovered later.

The elevators came directly up to the nurse's closed-in desk, and there were a few benches to sit on. This was where we spent most of our visitation time. We were observed through the glass of the nurses' desk.

As it turned out, the hospital professionals were rude and disinterested. Beth told me she was frightened of them. They thought she was faking her illness and told me so. Their expectations were greater for her than she could handle. She was unable to read their directives or rules. A pamphlet of rules had been given to her, and she tried desperately to read it. Sadly, and in frustration, she said, "Mom, I can't read it!"

One day, they told her she could not see Kyle since she didn't get up on time. (This was one of the rules she was to observe from the pamphlet.) She was crushed and called me to ask me not to bring the baby. She became rather hysterical, because she was afraid I would bring Kyle and the staff would be angry. Her psychiatrist had given instructions that she could see her baby every day. She was too confused to remember his words and too afraid to disobey the staff. I suspect the communication between physician and staff could have been much improved.

In the first two weeks of her hospitalization, Beth could not remember which of her clothes were clean and which were not. She frequently sent home clean clothes. Her hair was messy, and her skin was blotchy. The paleness seemed to be more pronounced. The staff allowed me to bring clothes and personal items.

(*Anecdotal: postpartum psychotic patients tend to become many shades lighter than their original skin tone. – James A. Hamilton, MD*)

She said, "Mom, I can't watch TV or look at magazines. It is too hard. People talk around me, and it confuses me." This was true even after she was released the first time. She could not hold a conversation of any length and seemed unable to finish a thought if someone made noise around us.

Beth slept much of the time, which annoyed the staff. She told me there was one nurse she really liked and who had been sympathetic to her. But that did not keep the others from trying to keep her up and moving. Perhaps there was a reason for this, but I did not understand it. After all, she was on heavy medication, and she was ill. They expected her to function normally: get up, get dressed, eat breakfast, go to classes...

Other patients took her things. The nurses were rude to both of us and used a superior and condescending tone with us, and they were often very sarcastic. It seemed as though they thought this was a hoax Beth was pulling, and it was not worth their time and assistance. There was no protection for her if I was not there. Some were heard saying, "She just wants attention." I was allowed to bring her clothes, but not to stay. We were all allowed to sit out in the lobby each night under the scrutiny of the nurses on duty.

At one time, someone had taken all her towels, and she had not taken a shower or washed her hair in three days. Beth told the staff, but nothing was done to remedy the situation.

"They told me to look in the linen area, Mom. I'll show you."

No towels were there. We approached her nurse and explained she needed towels. The nurse would not look at or speak to me.

He said, "Now Beth, you know there are towels in that room." He called her a liar. I noticed she was having trouble explaining, and I tried to explain.

He angrily said to me, "Beth will have to ask me if she wants anything."

So they looked and found no towels. She was told to wait. Beth could not stay focused on anything long enough to actually speak to him or ask any questions. It was so obvious; I couldn't imagine that this nurse could not comprehend. I was asked to leave.

I was not sure whether all of her problems were from the psychosis or the medication. They had begun treating her with anti-depressants during this time.

Out of frustration, I took her little "rule book" and wrote "I love you" here and there throughout the whole thing. I didn't know if she would even see it, but she was able to tell me much later that she read them. She thanked me, and I was so glad my idea worked out. I would recommend it in similar situations.

Each evening, we dressed Kyle and spent time at the hospital. It was hard to see her locked in there, but they allowed her to come out in the hall to sit with us and hold Kyle. Sometimes she didn't want to hold him. Sometimes she was indifferent and could have been holding any inanimate object. There were times when she wanted one of us to hold him.

My parents came from Minnesota and were in total denial when they visited her. But my stepfather told me how his first wife changed after their second child was born. He was unable to return to see Beth.

Chapter 7

Treatment

We had been were told the psychosis was not connected with the birth. The psychiatrist was quite adamant about it. She was medicated with an anti-depressant, imiprimine, and low doses of thyroid. It was not successful. After the tenth day, Mike and I were called in to talk to a specialist about electroconvulsive (ECT) therapy. Beth was very uncomfortable with the idea and cried softly. Beth had not been crying since she was hospitalized, at least not when we were there. The situation was difficult, and I was concerned about her frame of mind. She said, "I'm afraid of this, Mom. What should I do?" We spent several hours in discussion with the doctor who was going to administer the therapy, and she finally made a decision to accept this alternative treatment. She remained frightened. She talked to me about it and sobbed, "I'm so scared, Mom." ECT was really our only alternative.

The idea of ECT was disturbing to me as well. She was becoming much worse. Beth seemed disconnected to everyone but me. Because I am epileptic, I tried to use it as an example so she would not be so afraid. I had trouble rationalizing that in my own mind. I explained to Beth that my seizures had not harmed me, and that helped her decide. The doctor explained, "This therapy is no longer as rigorous as most people are led to believe. We now use drugs to prevent movement under anesthetic." That helped. She seemed calmer.

Mike and I arrived at the hospital for each session of ECT, rode the elevator down with her, and waited for her. The nurses were rude and told us we had no right to ride in these elevators, because they were for hospital personnel only. It didn't stop us! We were angry. Each time she returned from a session, the difference was remarkable. Beth was animated and happy. She smiled and moved quickly. She seemed much closer to her real self. It was a wonderful change! "I feel really good," she exclaimed. But it never lasted very long. She had her fourth and last therapy just before Christmas. She had been in the hospital since December 10, 1986.

The ECT was abruptly discontinued. Why? What happened? Did they feel it was not working? We were not told. Much later I was to discover the reason, described by Dr. Jones as a "bad reaction." He said that she was "speaking in tongues." The staff had informed him of this. He admitted he knew nothing of this "speaking in tongues" and later explained she had been speaking gibberish for several hours. Dr. James Hamilton, a specialist in the area of postpartum illnesses, later told me he felt they quit too soon. He said that since they were looking for a change, they should have acknowledged this and continued.

(Today, we know that ECT is effective if handled properly. For some, it is much better than medications.)

Chapter 8

First Release

Beth was allowed to go home overnight after that final therapy session. It was nearly Christmas, and my parents were quite excited to see her. We were happy she was released, but felt she was still very sick. She wanted me or Mike to make all her decisions.

My parents were still here from Minnesota, and her brother Jim and his wife, Cindee, arrived from Florida. We decided to have an early Christmas celebration and keep things on the quiet side, but Beth wanted to go to sleep right after dinner. She seemed to need a lot of sleep. When she was awakened, she was confused and upset. It didn't really make any sense to the family.

Jim, her brother, was traumatized. Jim had been away for quite a while, so this was the first time he saw her in this state. It was his first glimpse of Kyle, too. He didn't know what to say, and when he tried to be himself (he was always joking with Beth), she reacted as if she did not understand and became agitated. He expected her to laugh at his jokes as she always did. She became frustrated instead and hid her face. Jim got his first real picture of psychosis. He began blaming himself for not coming sooner. Beth had called him many times, he told us. I guess we all were accepting our share of guilt and blame. The Christmas presents remained untouched. Unable to cope with conversation, she asked to go home. Mike took her back to the hospital in the morning.

My parents were still visiting after Christmas when Beth was suddenly released from the hospital. They were thrilled and thought she was well. Soon they began to ask questions about her behavior and some of the nonsense things she said. She had come directly here from the hospital with Mike. I felt it was too early to release her, based on her inability to solve problems and her lack of short-term memory. It seemed like the Christmas fiasco should have told the doctor she was not fit to be alone. I was never given a chance to voice any of these opinions, because parents are not told anything about their adult married child. The husband is the only one the physician addresses. Actually, no one told Mike much of anything.

She was unable to decide what to do next, how to organize, or to plan a small gathering for Kyle's baptism. She told me that she realized she shouldn't have been released yet. She did not seem to understand or be able to cope. But Beth seemed happier, and she smiled. She told me her private reason for wanting out of the hospital was to get Kyle baptized. I am convinced she was able to fool the doctor and the staff – at least for a short time. She had been there for most of a month.

It was as if she feared not to have him baptized immediately. She seemed to have a lot of disturbing thoughts concerning her religious beliefs. During the baptism in early January, she handed Kyle to Jim to hold. Jim was Kyle's Godfather. Baptism was essential to our faith, but there was never a rush about having the service.

(*I later attributed her anxiousness about having an early baptism to fear of harming him. This is not unusual in a psychosis. Many have religious ideas incongruent with their earlier beliefs. Some think the baby is the devil, some think they are the devil, some are totally out of balance about all of this. You can see how a suicide or infanticide might occur.*)

In early January, I had to make the arrangements for the baptismal party because Beth still seemed unable to handle it. I was happy to be able to do something for her. She was able to call the pastor and arrange a date. Her concentration was so poor that she forgot whom she invited, unintentionally forgot to ask special friends, and the party was held at my house. I didn't want her to think I didn't trust her, so I did ask her to bring the punch. Mike followed through with that. Beth seemed very happy and enjoyed the day.

Chapter 9

Back Again

A week later, Beth called me and said, "Guess where I'm going?" She was going back to the hospital. "Do you want me to come?" "Yes," she said. So I went along with her, Mike, and Kyle. It was a beautiful sunny day. They accepted her as if she was a nuisance. The attitude was pervasive.

Hospitalization lasted all of January and most of February of 1987. Her mental health was not much better. Her skin was blotchy from her medications, and she seemed unable to express herself. I was glad to see her return because she needed the help and suicide watch. I hoped the hospital staff would know what to do. Was this ever going to end? I worried about how it might end in suicide. I prayed to God often for strength to do the right things to help Beth through this psychosis and to give her peace. She was my baby and always would be. Both Mike and Kyle spent this hospitalization time at our house, at her request.

I would have gladly taken her place and endured this psychosis if I could have. Nothing is worse than watching your child suffer and being unable to stop it.

The situation was becoming worse. Would this never be right? Beth was imprisoned by her own mind. Our lives became days of terror. Her speech was slow. She looked drugged. She clung to me, and I knew I had to be very careful not to make decisions for her. Nothing was going well. She once told her dad, "Kyle is purple tonight." So she still had hallucinations or delusions. She was gaining weight, perhaps from the medication. Her coloring was not good. I saw her walk was slow and unusual, and it was difficult to talk to her. She looked very sad all the time.

It was early February when the psychologist decided to help. He asked Mike's parents, Mike, Dave and I to attend a meeting with him and Beth. It was to be at his convenience, and we were told if even one of us could not come, this meeting would not take place. Every one of us made an effort to comply.

We gathered in this sterile-looking room and took chairs in a small circle. Another psychologist arrived. The purpose of the meeting was to construct a helpful plan for Beth. He began by telling

Beth, "Please go around the room and tell each person here how you have inconvenienced them by your hospital stay. You may begin with Mike."

I was ready to leave right then. Imagine, thinking she was responsible! She stammered through this, and I thought she was extremely cooperative. She did want to leave the hospital, so she did what she was told. We all looked very uncomfortable, and I know I was. Everyone was upset and angry but didn't know what to do. We discussed this later, out of her sight. Whatever his objective, I knew it was not psychologically sound. I have taken a number of psychology courses, taught school, raised four children, and have also seen several psychologists to deal with my own problems or those of my children, so I feel I have some knowledge about this. The only reason I stayed was because I did not want to upset Beth.

They gave us no plan whatsoever! But they expected us to come back for a second time. I said "no" to that. No help was given the first time. Beth was blamed for everything. The psychologist said to me, "There will be no more meetings if you do not come. You will ruin it for Beth." He didn't seem to understand Beth or me. I came to the conclusion no one realized **she was afraid of herself and what she might do to Kyle.** Later, Dr. Jones and some of the staff admitted they had not understood. Beth didn't seem to care about these meetings, nor did she understand their purpose when we talked. She later said it did not matter to her, and she had expressed a strong dislike of this psychologist from the first week she was there.

(*I would like to interject that I, too, was seeing the psychiatrist for several reasons. Mainly, I wanted to find out what was happening with Beth. Psychiatrists are not at liberty to give out information directly to parents of married women. I had known Dr. Jones before, and this was the only way to be able to understand what was happening from his point of view. The second reason was that I needed all the help I could get in order to deal with this devastating psychosis. Thirdly, since Beth had put so much weight on everything I said or did, I wanted some guidance. I continued to see Dr. J. until well after her death.*)

In mid-February, I had to go out of town for a few days. While I was away, some "staff" at the hospital decided Beth needed "mothering skills." During that time, Kyle was brought to her, and she was placed in a hospital room alone with a bottle, diapers, formula, and a playpen. There were two beds, and the playpen was between them. There were two hospital chairs. It was a colorless room in grays and greens. Bottles, formula, and diapers were placed on one bed, and warm water was available for formula from the bathroom. She had not taken care of this baby for three months. How was she supposed to do it now? This was not an educational experience! Beth was totally petrified when this happened. She shared this with me later that day. This appeared to be very traumatic for her, because when I arrived home, she was on the phone with Mike begging him to come for Kyle. ***She had been set up for failure***.

She was so depressed; she told Mike she didn't want to see us. We went right over, because I knew she needed us. I was right. At the locked ward, the nurse told us Beth didn't want any guests. But I saw her standing back behind the nurses' office through the glass. She told them to unlock the doors. I watched her walk to her room, climb into bed with all her clothes on, and pull the covers over her head as she sobbed. It was so awful and frightening. They never understood that Beth did not need mothering skills; she needed a lot of medical help. It was like something out of a bad movie.

Beth had been babysitting for most of her life. When she was 15, she took care of her brother's young baby, Aaron, in Texas for a whole summer. She had always loved children and felt very comfortable about caring for them. For many years, she would appear at the organ after church carrying a little baby. She always said, "Isn't this the cutest baby you have ever seen?" The doctors and staff had never figured out that **she was afraid of herself–afraid she might hurt her little baby.**

Was I angry and frustrated? YES! And very afraid! It is beyond my comprehension that all those "professionals" could not understand. The staff and Dr. Jones later on told me they realized this mistake. I sincerely hope that it is one mistake they will never repeat.

Her hospital confinement continued until late February–approximately three months. Once she told me, "Mom, I asked to be locked up in the back ward."

This is the isolation area. She refused to say why when I asked. Shortly after the "experiment" of having Kyle there, Beth began to call me and say:

"I want to go home," or

"I can never remember what I was going to say to the doctor," or

"What can I do?"

She told me she could not remember what to say to her doctor until the time he came each day. She asked repeatedly about what she should say. Her speech was much slower than earlier and almost inaudible. I asked her what she wanted to say, and she slowly told me:

"I hate the hospital. No one, no one cares about me."

"I want to come home and be with Mike."

"I am tired of this place and think I would be better off at home."

"No one listens to me."

"I am not getting better."

47

I told her I could not take the responsibility of telling the hospital what she thought. I urged her to make her own decision. I really hoped she would be able to ask to leave on her own.

I so badly wanted to run over to the hospital and grab her in my arms and bring her home with me. But it was impossible!

Later in the day, she would call again and ask the same questions. She was clearly unhappy.

"Mom, I left the ward today and was gone for over an hour. I went all over the hospital and down to the restaurant in the basement. No one asked me where I had been, and they opened the doors and let me back in. Honestly, Mom, they are not watching me. I know no one will believe me. I don't think they care."

Beth thought I wouldn't believe her, so she repeated it. How she did it was a mystery. She had a roommate who left each day to feed her cat, and I suppose Beth left with the roommate. Her absence was never reported.

Beth kept saying, "They don't want me here. They don't care about me. I would be safer at home." I also felt they considered her a bother, as I observed the way they ignored her and avoided her. She had been there too long.

A staff member said, "Beth really isn't sick at all."

During her hospital stay, Mike lost his job. He was not visibly concerned and said, "I can always get another job." Because he wasn't going to a job each day, it seemed logical Beth would be safer at home. I don't think Beth felt comfortable about their loss of income, and it was one more factor contributing to the illness.

(Psychosocial issues such as grief factors add to this problem. Loss of wages, the hospitalization, loss of insurance benefits, and the illness itself are types of grief factors.)

She was finally able to tell her doctor she wanted to go home. It took her several days, since she had no short-term memory. Dr. Jones told her he was angry and blamed it on me. I didn't care. It was her decision! She was much better off at home. She knew she wasn't well, but managed. She rarely held Kyle then.

Needless to say, our whole family was grappling with anger, lack of understanding, sorrow, guilt, and disbelief when faced with a psychosis we had never seen before in our happy, outgoing, strong Beth.

Chapter 10

Home

Out of the clear blue, Beth suddenly got better. **It was almost April, and she was a lot better**! She went to the hairdresser, bought baby clothes, cooked, and enjoyed Kyle a great deal. She said she knew she was better, but was not entirely well. But she seemed rational again. Her brother, Michael, was getting married in Texas in April. She did not plan to go, but called him several times. She told Michael, "I'm so happy for you, and I'm sorry I won't be able to come, but I'm not quite well." We were thrilled to get our real Beth back.

(Many times when psychosis seems to be disappearing, it is a clue to watch carefully. I have been told this by many moms who experienced psychosis. They all told me when they felt really good, then something bad happened and they had a setback.)

Beth and I went shopping for a new hat for Kyle. We couldn't find what we wanted. He had a very "funny looking" hat, and we had laughed about that. We had a Coke at Burger King, and a young mother and baby walked by the window. She started to laugh and said, "And you think my baby has a funny hat! Look at that one!" It was decidedly worse than Kyle's hat and indeed funny. We giggled for quite a while over our Cokes.

The "good time" lasted about two weeks. Suddenly it was as if it **were the day I took her to the hospital**. She told me, "I know I was well last week, but I can't even remember what that felt like." Beth always had a cat and was very comforted by her cat, Whisper. But now I watched her put him into the garage instead of allowing him to sit in her lap. *How unusual!* I thought to myself.

She was so miserable, and so was I. I suggested she return to her doctor and talk with him at length. She did. She also reported he had not taken her seriously. It turned out she was right. Later I was to find out she told him she was suicidal. His reaction was, "I didn't think Beth was **actively** suicidal." I couldn't even respond to that!

Some unusual things happened in Beth's life that last week. She was frightened by a tall raggedy street man who walked into our church service on Palm Sunday, and he moved to the front of the church. His hands were held up high in the air. It surprised everyone.

51

He was not known by anyone in our congregation and was following our pastor to the altar where he lay down on the steps with arms outstretched shouting, "Hallelujah, Hallelujah!" It was spooky to us, but very scary for Beth. Our pastor was able to get him into a seat, but he left as abruptly as he had arrived. Beth talked about it constantly. I got the impression that she felt it was some kind of warning from God.

During that same week, Beth began visiting friends, with Mike of course. I thought it unusual that she didn't wait for people to come to see Kyle. After being ill for so long, it seemed out of context. I now think she was saying, "Good-bye."

Easter was approaching, and Beth was a member of the Bell Choir, along with her dad. In spite of her depression, he said to her, "I will pick you up for early church. It might make you feel better to play the bells." They both rang bells at both services on Easter. She always loved ringing bells. She had bought a new jumper and borrowed a blouse from me. I offered her an Easter cross to wear, and she was adamant about saying "No!" *Strange, but maybe she is trying to be independent*, I thought. Later, I realized there was a religious connection she was avoiding. She played flawlessly, and they went to Mike's family for dinner.

We were not aware that the conversation that Easter Sunday was about asphyxiation due to carbon monoxide gas. She apparently kept asking about it, as it was in the paper that day. We also didn't know she had asked for a gun, and that Mike had hidden anything in the house or garage that he felt could have harmed her.

We went to see Beth and Mike at their house in the evening. She was holding Kyle and looked much better. When we left, she protested. "Do you HAVE to go?" This was unusual. Dad said, "I have to get home for my insulin." So I kissed her, and we left. I can still see her sitting in the big rocker, holding Kyle, and trying to smile. She really did look better. I guess we were fooling ourselves.

THAT WAS THE LAST TIME I SAW HER ALIVE!

Chapter 11

Death as an Answer?

Easter night, my mother called and wanted to know how Beth was doing. I told Mom that Beth was really slipping down again, and what had happened during the previous few days. Mom became angry with me and accused me of spending too much time at Beth and Mike's house, and not minding my own business. She said, "You are not giving Beth a chance to resume her own responsibilities, and you should stay away for a while. "You can't live her life for her, and you are just making it worse than it really is."

Needless to say, Mom hit below the belt. She really didn't understand what was happening, and I am sure she was very afraid. There was no use explaining again, so we ended the conversation. I'm now sorry that I didn't listen to my own heart, because I decided to give Beth one day without my presence. I guess mothers influence their children, even into adulthood. It was probably not a wise decision on my part – but how can you really know? It was to be one thing I regretted for many years.

On Monday evening, I couldn't stand it any longer and asked Dave to call and see how she was doing. She sounded so depressed and told him she couldn't feed Kyle. I was determined to get down there on Tuesday. I had an organ lesson in the morning and a lot of phone calls and interruptions when I got home. Then the phone rang! It was a strange-sounding Mike, saying, "Get down here! Get down here!" So I got in my car, leaving the house unlocked, and drove the few miles south to their house.

All the way I was trying not to think. I would say to myself,

"Is it Beth?" or
"Is it Kyle" or
"Is it both?"
"No, it can't be! It just can't be!"
"Maybe it isn't too bad."
"Maybe I'll be there in time."
"Did she harm Kyle?"
"Did she have an accident?"

"No! No! No!"

I didn't want to think about it. The windows of the car were wide open and the wind and heat were all around me. I didn't care. I turned off my feelings as much as I could.

"No, I can't think like that. God, please help ME! God, please help Beth!"

I was praying for things to turn out right all the way. I didn't even want to consider suicide.

It was the longest few miles I ever drove. I talked myself into total denial about anything that could have happened. But when I pulled up into the driveway, I saw her lying on the garage floor. She was wearing navy blue sweatpants and a white T-shirt and her sweatpants were wet. What had happened? She couldn't be dead! Why was I so frightened then? I was numb. But I didn't think she was dead. **I didn't want to think she was dead! I couldn't speak!**

Mike and his neighbor were giving her CPR. The Rescue Squad had been called and was arriving. Mike hailed the Rescue Squad and told me to take over. I had never taken CPR and was petrified! But I had seen it often on TV, and Beth demonstrated it when she was a member of the Rescue Squad. So I did my best. I had been holding her hand and her fingernails were bluish. I thought, "This is a bad sign." When I breathed into her, a strange noise came out. I still hadn't given up, though. The Rescue Squad, police, and ambulances arrived. There were many people. Beth had been an EMT with the Squad for eight years, and they all showed their loyalty and caring.

Mike and I were chased into the house by the medics. They had the "paddles" in their hands and were cutting her shirt. It seemed like such a personal invasion; I tried to stay. They closed the door in my face. Mike was wailing and calling to God. I remember telling myself that I couldn't afford to get out of control. I couldn't help crying some. I was still denying this whole scene.

Since I did not know what had happened, I checked the medicine bottles. All pills were accounted for. My stomach was churning. Mike offered to help me.

I called Dave at work. Mike had tried to call there earlier, but did not reach Dave. Feelings were running rampant, but I had to keep calm. I just had to! Since Dave could not be reached, I left a message. I began to feel panic. Next, I called the church. Our organist, Linda, answered the phone and said our pastor was away. It seems most of the Lutheran pastors in town were away. I didn't want to think about death. In spite of what I wanted to believe, I still told Linda, "Beth is dead." But I neglected to tell her where we were. I still didn't know what had happened to Beth. It was not obvious.

Kyle awoke, and a neighbor was heating a bottle. I don't even remember when she came into the house. Kyle was 5 months old. I went to him, and he gave me the biggest grin a baby could give. It was so ironic–a happy little baby who didn't know he had no mother. I really started to cry then. I had been holding it back but that smile was so innocent.

Mike was waiting for me to go to the hospital, and the ambulance driver refused me entry. Mike said we would take my car, and he would drive. I got in. It wasn't until we were driving to the hospital that Mike told me **she hung herself with a jump rope**. Shock! Disbelief! Deep Sadness! Now what was I to do, and how was I going to get through it? How were we all to understand and work through this terrible disaster? My baby, my poor little Beth was gone! I had a great feeling of despair, shock and helplessness. I wanted her back!!

The hospital said, "They're working on her." This couldn't be true, as they had put her in the ambulance at least a half an hour earlier and would let no one near her. I was angered by the statement and wondered what they were trying to keep from me. The chaplain took us to a small room. Suddenly, I had to go into the bathroom where I could get away. It was chaotic. I wanted to see her. I couldn't bear to remember her on the garage floor. Mike told me on the way to the hospital that he had gone for a job interview for an hour, and that was when she had hung herself. He said she had seemed so much better and had urged him to leave.

Mike's family and friends arrived. I felt alone, even though we were in the same room. Pastor B. arrived for me. He was a former pastor to us and had married Beth and Mike. I still wanted to see Beth and told them, "If you do not make arrangements immediately for me to see Beth, I will find her myself!" The chaplain took me back. She was so peaceful. She was so beautiful. All I could do was hug her and tell her I loved her and cry. I really wanted to be alone with her, but that was not possible. So many people.

Soon Dave arrived. The message Mike had sent earlier had been confused, and he had gone home instead of to Beth's house. When he didn't find me at our home, he went to Beth and Mike's house and found a policeman making a report. That was when he was told we had gone to the hospital. It wasn't until he arrived that I told him Beth was dead. He said, "Poor Beth," and began to cry.

Pastor B. drove me home in my car, and Dave drove his. The pastor's wife came soon after that, and they stayed a while. Eventually, he assisted with the funeral service, along with our own pastor.

I remember sitting on the floor with Dave, calling our parents and three boys. My mother screamed, and Dave's mother wept. The boys tried to be strong, but were very shaken. After the phone calls and more tears, we said, "Where is everyone? Someone should be here for us." A knock came at the door. It was a group of friends from church. We were saved momentarily.

Life was a blur for a while. We managed to get through the funeral and greet people. I don't remember much of it. The line at the funeral home was blocks long, and I do remember hugging a lot people and crying. The boys were home and definitely frazzled. There is something called "denial" that helps you cope. She was buried in a beautiful cemetery under a large water oak she had admired. That was only the beginning of a different life for all of us.

(Beth did not fit the profile for any risk factors for postpartum depression or psychosis, except severe PMS. She had a good solid support system of family and friends, and there was no hereditary factor for mental illness in the family. Her relationship with her parents and husband was delightful, and she had no physical problems, no abuse, no drugs, and no alcohol. She had the ability to deal with childcare and a love for children. She had no fear of coping with small babies. I have learned that psychosis can occur even without risk factors. But we now know it is wise to ask questions about these factors to try and prevent possible suicides in the future. Fortunately, new medications are now available and new therapies as well.)

Chapter 12

The Truly Understanding Pastor

A person completes commits suicide when they become hopeless, helpless, and hapless. They feel they have nowhere else to turn. *"Suicide" is not the result of one moment or one wound. It is a slow accumulation of pain often triggered by a physical malady." – from* Preventing Suicide, <u>National Journal,</u> *March/April 2003.*

Our pastor had great insight into Beth's illness, even though others thought differently. He saw her at the hospital daily and knew her well. So I am sharing excerpts of his kind words from the funeral sermon on April 24, 1987.

"...We are not here to turn away or to pretend it didn't happen or it doesn't matter. We are here to ask questions and try to understand...

"...sometimes the motive is our own. We see death as our choice, the solution to problems, a way of getting back at someone, an alternative to facing life, and we calculate and rationally take our own life.

"But Beth had no rational motive. She had no reason. In fact, she had every reason not to die. She had a child, a husband, a family, friends, a whole church that loved her. She did not die because of motives, hers or anyone else's. And her death was not an accident. And that leaves DISEASE – not of the heart, but of another even more complex organ, the brain. Her mind was not functioning as it should – Beth had no control. She died of a disease, a mental disorder, which for her was terminal.

"...had her death been an accident...or whatever, the tragedy of it would be no less great – nor more. Our pain would be the same...we still look for answers.

"Looking at Beth's faith – a faith clearly evidenced by her regularity at worship and in Sunday School, and by her service in this place where as a member of our Handbell Choir, she contributed so much to the worship of so many of us – looking at her obvious faith...

"...the heart of God aches with his Son's, and our, tragedy. He feels it even more than we do. AND WHILE NEITHER BETH

NOR THE DOCTORS NOR YOU NOR I HAVE ANY CONTROL OVER DEATH, HE DOES!

"We haven't stopped loving Beth. Do we think the very creator of life himself who lifted up his own Son and led him from the tomb has? Of course not!

"...but Christ's cross was made the key to unlock both the door of the tomb and gate of heaven for all the faithful – and that means for Beth."

We all found these words very comforting!

My question suddenly became, "How does this Man of God know what her doctor doesn't even understand?" Perhaps I will never have an answer to that, but I am grateful for the understanding he gave me.

Chapter 13

Was It A Dream?

That I really held you in my arms and sang lullabies to you, touching your soft cheek against mine?

That I watched you take your first steps to your Daddy?

That I watched you walk to kindergarten alone and independent, not wanting to see you grow up, as I carefully followed you all the way?

That I attended your first ballet recital, and was excited to learn that you had won an award?

That you grew into a young lady when I saw you in your prom gown? So beautiful!

That you actually agreed to play a clarinet duet with me in church, just to please me?

You were the most beautiful bride in the world.

You shared your love with everyone.

You always had time for us, calling to check on our whereabouts, appearing suddenly to cheer us up, offering everything of yourself.

It seems like so long ago when you were here to make us so happy! We all still miss you! We always will!

Chapter 14

Coping With Suicide, Loss of a Child

Losing a child is the most difficult thing anyone has to face. We needed help. Crying, blaming ourselves, and seeing her in everyone else, was hard to face. But the hardest was looking into the face of little Kyle and seeing Beth. They looked so much alike, it was amazing. Knowing he would never know his mother was traumatic. His first birthday hit me like a ton of bricks, knowing his mother should be here for him but would never be.

We were unable to live our usual lifestyle. We were unable to function, buy groceries, pay bills, weed the yard, keep track of whether we ate or not, and we were unable to sleep. Great waves of tears struck us frequently and without warning.

We received a letter from The Compassionate Friends and decided to go to their meeting. This is where we found sharing friends and lots of love. Going to meetings was not as easy as we thought. I became very stubborn about the whole idea and claimed I would not speak at the first meeting. Then I was welcomed by a mother of one of my eighth grade students, a son who was accidentally killed by his friend during the time I was his teacher. I talked a lot and cried all the while.

At the second meeting, I refused to get out of the car. I finally changed my mind, because Dave was upset and began roaming the dark sidewalks near the car. After that, it was a little easier. I guess you realize by now how stubborn I am. Eventually, we both learned that this was a comfort place where you could be yourself and get support.

But suicide death is different to deal with than death from illness or accidents. We met a couple who were also suffering and wanted to start a group for anyone who was dealing with suicide. We started a group called "Touched By Suicide." It was very helpful and time-consuming, and it halved our grief. Sharing was so important. Our group still exists and has helped many over these sixteen years. **Our faith in God, our congregation, and our support groups are primary factors in healing.**

Reading the obituary of your child in the newspapers makes you feel as if this little piece of paper couldn't possibly tell anyone who my daughter is. It is as if her whole life was reduced to a few sentences. And I remember thinking about flowers and how they, too, would soon be as dead as Beth in a couple of days. Later, I had to realize that mourners are not with you after a few weeks in any way. They are thinking you should just "get over it." If only it were that easy.

And no one will ever know just how far-reaching the grief ripples travel to other friends, and especially relatives, who knew and loved Beth. My mother finally understood and believed what I had tried to explain. And how could I help my other children, who all lived in different states?

Our youngest son, Mike, sought help immediately from his pastor. He was able to talk about Beth and what happened, and eventually get some resolve.

Our middle son, Jim, stayed in denial for almost fifteen years. He was not totally himself during this time, made some bad decisions, and refused to tell people what happened or share Beth's story. He finally went to get some professional help, and I am happy to say he has dealt with all of this. He is now a happy person again.

Our eldest son, Gary, seemed to turn himself off from all of the thoughts concerning Beth. He didn't want to talk about it to anyone and only mentioned her on her death date. We had two very brief discussions until he read this book and got the whole picture. He had not asked specifically what happened. I think he is working toward acceptance now.

Worrying about how your children are coping is a big thing. They all lived in different states, and we did not see them often. They were wonderful about sending cards, calling, and inviting us to their homes for holidays. But they really didn't want to discuss death with us. They were worried about upsetting us.

It would be impossible to explain the depth of emotion involved in this grieving process. And contrary to what most people are taught, it is impossible to even begin dealing with this for about 2 years. Grieving takes its toll on health as well. I spent the first two years with multiple illnesses, surgery, heart problems and broken bones. Eventually, my immune system stopped working temporarily.

About five months after her death, I began to sink into a deep depression. I didn't want to leave the house, see friends, or move about, and would have liked to have been left completely alone. I recognized this as depression. Knowing it and doing something about it are two different things.

I did not take any medications. I began to think about what would happen if I took my own life. It eventually became clear to me that I couldn't consider suicide because I knew what happened to all of us and our friends and relatives as a result of losing Beth. I began to think about Kyle and Dave and our children. Little by little, things began to look better. I knew I had to do this myself, so I did the best I could. Eventually, the depression went away…slowly. Dave talked with me and helped me decide to get better.

I started to do some writing for myself as a way to deal with the death. In October, I wrote this note to Beth. October is her birth month.

Dearest Beth – my baby,

When I remember you, the tears won't stop. Just to see you, touch you, hold you and love you one more time would be heavenly. But I could not say goodbye then either. The pain of your absence is too great! I must choose to live this existence on earth without you in the knowledge of our reunion in the next life.

You have been my best friend who loves me at any cost. You have warmed me with the sunshine of your smile and the pleasure of your laughter. You have caused me great pain but brought me more love.

70

I miss our sharing...and caring...because you were always there for me.

In May I wrote again.

I needed to talk to you today, Beth, but I couldn't. It seems so long since I've held you or even seen you. I miss you just as much as always.

Mother's Day is coming up, and all the TV ads are showing special mother-daughter stories. It makes me sad not to have you here. You always made me feel so special and important. You were always so sweet and loving.

Kyle is here with me this week. He is such a darling boy—so much like you were at that age. I feel sad he will never know you and that you are not here to see him grow.

He has your wonderful sense of humor and laughs at Dad's puns.

He calls me "Honey," and loves grandpa's tools in the garage. He eats green beans and broccoli. He helps set the table and makes up words like "all the where" for everywhere. He loves your kitty Jasmine and was hugging her this morning. You would be so proud of him.

I love you so much! I hope God takes good care of you!

Love and kisses, forever, Mom

(The first time I went to the grocery store after her death, I began to reach for one of her favorite foods. Then the reality set in–I didn't need it anymore! This thought sent me into tears on the spot.)

Grieving is so difficult, because it is hard work, and no one else can do it for you. Even though you and your spouse have the same loss, it isn't really the same. Everyone has their own way of handling it, and it depends on the relationship you had with the person.

The depression was only temporary, fortunately. The emotional shock will never leave, and **our love for Beth remains forever**. We will always miss her!

Chapter 15
Kyle's Help

Kyle was a saving grace for me. I knew he needed care, and I knew how to give it. He became so very precious and turned out to be a very easy baby. I cut my crying significantly when he was here, and he was here often in those first few years. It was such fun to play with him, read to him, take him to the park, to preschool, to the lake, or just to love him. And Dave had just as much fun with Kyle. I had never played in a large box before, spent time in Toys R Us, crawled in and out of tents and tiny play houses, learned how to swing again under the magnolia tree, and played a host of games I didn't know existed. Eventually he would ask me, "Are you going to cry today, Honey?" I was able to answer with a, "no."

Kyle is now a senior in high school, working toward becoming an Eagle Scout, crucifer at church, and a member of both the wind ensemble and the Honors Band. He is a member of the National Honor Society and a loving grandson. We are very proud of him. He also plays in Bell Choir, like Beth. Kyle seems to like art, symphonies, ballet, plays, movies, friends, school, and his grandparents. He tells people that we think he is perfect. And we do think that. It will be difficult to have him away at school next year.

Kyle's father remarried Lori when he was four years old, and he has two younger half-brothers named Corey and Connor. They seem to think a lot of their older brother, and he loves them. The family lives about 30 minutes from us, near Kyle's high school. We see them in church every Sunday, and we are all good friends.

Dave and I try to provide educational events that would be difficult for Mike. We take him on trips across the USA, Canada, and Mexico. We take him to the symphony, plays, Sunday lunches, Festival of Trees (where his mother's name is always displayed at Christmas), and to visit Beth's brothers in Texas, Washington, and a number of other areas where they have lived. He has ties to my family in Iowa, and Dave's family in Minnesota, where we make regular visits. He was well-traveled by the time he was four years old.

Kyle dearly loved his first trip to the farm in Iowa. He liked the tractor rides, the 4-H fairs, the cows, and the timbers where we rode the hay wagon. We finished that trip off with a visit to Dave's family on a northern Minnesota lake. He was fascinated to be able to see the small fish clearly and lay on the dock for long periods of time watching them.

How to tell Kyle about his mother was a problem. He taught us instead. When he was three years old, I went to pick him up from pre-school. He had just begun to realize others were being picked up by mothers. He was usually picked up by "Honey," his name for me. When I arrived he said, "I want to see my Mommy!"

I always wore a locket with Beth's picture inside, and I gave it to him. He opened it and said to the children who were all sitting around a table waiting, "This is my Mommy! See, I do have a Mommy!"

They asked, "Where is she?"

"She is in Heaven with God," he replied.

"Oh," was the answer, and it was obvious they were calm. Then one boy asked, "Why is she in Heaven?"

"She was very sick and died," Kyle replied.

"Okay," was the response, and that was the end of the conversation. Isn't it wonderful how children are so accepting? The question never came up again with these children.

When Kyle was 10, we explained what had happened to his mother and why. Well, as much as we could. We felt he could deal in abstracts by then. Children think in concrete ideas when they are small. They're kind of "what you see is what it is" about things. But he does understand and had great feelings for children in his school that had learning problems or were handicapped. He accepted it well and asked a few questions. We told him he could ask about it at any given time. We would always be there for him.

Kyle is very much aware of postpartum depression and postpartum psychosis. He has hung around with me a lot and played quietly while I spent time with postpartum moms, just reassuring them. He is empathetic and understanding of them.

It is said that in death there is always a gift. What a hard concept to believe in. But it is true if you only look hard enough. Our gift came through the involvement in seeking answers concerning postpartum psychosis and depression, and in helping others. It continues to be so and always will.

Beth did not die of suicide. She died of a horrible disease. Because of her death, others have been helped. That is the joy that comes out of disaster. We are deeply grateful for the 25 years we enjoyed Beth and for the 16-plus years we have enjoyed Kyle, who is so much like her. We have many beautiful memories. She now enjoys the peacefulness and love of God in His great Heaven where we will someday be with her forever.

Chapter 16

So What Did I Learn?

Epilogue

The experience of living through a case of postpartum psychosis and following up with proper education taught me a lot. So I share with you what I can. If you are facing a similar situation, maybe something in this book will help you. You should be aware that psychosis has a biological basis. In other words, she cannot help that she is sick. Women are very susceptible to mental illness during and after pregnancy.

Psychosis is a horrible experience for both the patient and the family. That is a given.

When psychosis strikes, it is difficult to identify. If there is any doubt, see that the patient finds a psychiatrist who can make an evaluation. Do not assume all physicians understand or have training in this area. So ask questions about his/her practice, how many patients she/he has treated, if he/she is a member of DAD, Inc. or PSI, and ask yourself if you have a good feeling about this doctor from what he/she has shared with you.

After the type of postpartum illness has been identified as psychosis, the patient must be hospitalized. The reasons are clear: possibility of suicide, infanticide, and need for more intense care.

Make sure this mom has no physical problems such as low or high thyroid levels. Ask the physician about it and make sure she is tested.

The psychiatrist will decide on medications to help her. There are several classes of medication that will be effective. Many are a result of research in the field of postpartum mental health. He/she will also decide on a method to reach a goal of recovery. Be supportive of this.

When the new mother is released from the hospital, follow up with psychological therapy with a trusted professional. **If there is difficulty in finding a professional, check with PSI, DAD, Inc. or your state coordinator.**

A support group may be available in your area. Check it out with the local hospitals, health departments, or your state coordinator. PSI and DAD coordinators are listed on those web sites. The advantage of support groups is important. This gives everyone a chance to communicate their feelings without judgment.

Find all the educational materials available to you and read them. There has been so much available since 1986. The psychotic patient will probably not be able to read. It is important for the caretakers and family to know what to expect and be supportive. This psychosis will not go away in a few weeks or a few months, so patience is required. Husbands and families need to know what they are dealing with. Education is the first line of defense. Eventually, you will be able to educate the new mom, too.

Don't be afraid to call in another physician or psychologist if things are not going well. We all have our differences and need to feel comfortable with our caretakers.

Above all, assure this new mother: **She is not alone!**
This is not her fault!
She will get better!

Resources

Organizations

Postpartum Support International

(805) 967-7636

www.postpartum.net

Telephone support, international directory, information, and annual conference.

Depression After Delivery

(800) 944-4PPD

www.depressionafterdelivery.com

Answering machine. Free packets to new moms. Telephone Support.

The Marce Society

PO Box 30853

London, England W120XG

www.marcesociety.com

International organization dedicated to scientific research on postpartum disorders.

Annual conference.

North American Society for Psychosocial OB/GYN

409 12th St SW

Washington, DC 20024-2188

(202) 863-1628

www.naspog.com

Annual conference.

NC Depression After Delivery

(910) 791-5731

www.behavenet.com/ncdad

State organization, provides information, contacts, and referrals in NC.

Web Sites

Center for Postpartum Health

www.posttpartumhealth.com

Daybreak Alliance

www.Daybreakalliance.org

Depression After Delivery, Inc.

www.depressionafterdelivery.com

Medlineplus Health Information

www.nlm.nih.gov/medlineplus/postpartumdepression.html

NC Depression After Delivery

www.behavenet.com/ncdad

Postpartum Depression Online Support group

www.ppdsupportpage.com

Postpartum Stress Center

www.postpartumstress.com/

In Illinois:

www.ppdil.org

In New York:

www.postpartum@aol.com

Online Service: Diana L Barnes

www.dlbarnes@postpartumhealth.com

BETH

Ruth Rhoden Craven Foundation Inc. (South Carolina)
www.ppdsupport.org

For Husbands:
www.postpartumdads.org

Books

Bennett, Shoshana & Pec Indman, *Beyond the Blues: Prenatal and Postpartum Depression,* San Jose, CA: Moodswings Press, 2002

Dunnewold, Ann, *Evaluation and Treatment of Postpartum Emotional Disorders.* Sarasota, FL: Professional Resource Press, 1997

Dunnewold, Ann, and Diane Sanford, *The Postpartum Survival Guide.* Oakland, CA: New Harbinger Press, 1994

Kleiman, Karen, *The Postpartum Husband*, Philadelphia, PA: Xlibris, 2000

Kleiman, Karen and Valerie Raskin, *This Isn't What I Expected,* New York: Bantam Books, 1994

Misri, Shaila, *Shouldn't I Be Happy?: Emotional Problems of Pregnant and Postpartum Women*, New York: Free Press, 1995

Raskin, Valerie, *When Words Are Not Enough: Women's Prescription for Depression and Anxiety*, New York: Broadway Books, 1997

Sebastian, Linda, *Overcoming Postpartum Depression and Anxiety*, Omaha: Addicus Books, 1998

Sichel, Deborah and Jeanne Driscoll, *Women's Moods*, New York: William Morrow and Co., 1999

About the Author

Shirley Cervene Halvorson is a retired teacher of music and mathematics and has been educating new mothers and families about postpartum mental illness since the death of her daughter as a result of postpartum psychosis 16 years ago.

As a member of both Depression After Delivery, Inc.(DAD) and Postpartum Support International (PSI) since 1987, she is also North Carolina Coordinator for Postpartum Support International. She is also founder of North Carolina Depression After Delivery and a member of the NC Perinatal Mental Health Committee.

She is the recipient of a service award from DAD and the Jane Honikman award from PSI. She has been a telephone contact person for both DAD and PSI for 15 years, assisting new mothers and families through the crisis of postpartum mental health.

Shirley writes postpartum materials for the NCDAD organization. She became certified in Assessment and Treatment from PSI in June, 2003.

www.ingramcontent.com/pod-product-compliance
Lightning Source LLC
Chambersburg PA
CBHW021546290526
45785CB00004BA/1748